RANSOM KHANYE

The Red Hot Remedy

The Ultimate Guide to Cayenne Pepper Benefits

Cover design by Ransom Khanye
All copyrights reserved.

To subscribe to the author's mailing list and receive a free ebook send an email to:
raniekaysbooks@gmail.com

ISBN:9798882953453

Also available on Amazon, about natural remedies, and by the same author:

1. **The Magic Oil: Unleashing the Power of Nature's Remedy - Castor Oil**
2. **The Magic Oil 2: More Castor Oil Miracles**
3. **Amazing Natural Remedies: Nature's Medicine Cabinet**
4. **101 Castor Oil Recipes for Health and Beauty: The Complete Guide to Castor Oil Remedies**
5. **The Root of Health: Ginseng**
6. **Garlic: Nature's Miracle Clove**

[Note: This book does not make claims to diagnose, treat, or cure any specific diseases or medical conditions. It is intended for informational purposes only and should not replace professional medical advice or treatment.]

FOREWORD

Welcome to "The Red Hot Remedy: The Ultimate Guide to Cayenne Pepper Benefits." In this groundbreaking book, we embark on a journey into the fiery world of cayenne pepper—a spice revered for its remarkable healing properties and centuries-old legacy.

As you turn these pages, you'll discover the transformative potential of cayenne pepper to invigorate your health and elevate your well-being. From its ancient roots to modern-day applications, cayenne pepper has captivated cultures worldwide with its potent effects on mind, body, and spirit.

Get ready to be inspired as we delve into the science behind cayenne pepper's power, exploring its ability to ignite metabolism, soothe ailments, and enhance vitality. Through engaging narratives and evidence-based insights, you'll unlock the secrets of this red-hot remedy and learn how to harness its full potential in your own life.

Whether you're seeking relief from pain, support for heart health, or simply a zestier approach to wellness, "The Red Hot Remedy" offers practical guidance and expert advice to help you achieve your goals. Get set to ignite your health and embark on a journey of discovery with cayenne pepper as your trusted companion.

Let us embark on this spicy adventure together—a journey fueled by passion, knowledge, and the transformative power of nature's red-hot remedy.

Warm regards,

Ransom Khanye

Contents

Chapter 1: Introduction to Cayenne Pepper: A Spice Steeped in History and Tradition

In the bustling markets of ancient civilizations, amidst the vibrant tapestry of spices and aromas, one fiery gem stood out among the rest—cayenne pepper. This humble yet potent spice has a rich history steeped in tradition and cultural significance, captivating the senses and capturing the hearts of countless generations.

Tracing its origins back to the tropical regions of Central and South America, cayenne pepper, also known as Capsicum annuum, has been cultivated for thousands of years by indigenous peoples. The vibrant red hue of its slender pods hinted at the fiery heat concealed within, sparking curiosity and intrigue among early inhabitants of the Americas.

As trade routes expanded and explorers ventured into uncharted territories, cayenne pepper found its way into the culinary and medicinal practices of distant lands. From the bustling markets of ancient Egypt to the opulent courts of medieval Europe, this exotic spice soon became a coveted commodity, prized for its bold flavor and purported healing properties.

Across cultures and continents, cayenne pepper found its place in a myriad of culinary delights, adding depth and complexity to dishes ranging from hearty stews to savory sauces. But its influence extended far beyond the realm of gastronomy, as healers and herbalists revered cayenne pepper for its potent medicinal properties.

In traditional medicine systems such as Ayurveda and Traditional Chinese Medicine (TCM), cayenne pepper was valued for its ability to stimulate digestion, improve circulation, and alleviate various ailments. It was believed to possess warming properties that invigorated the body and restored balance to the mind and spirit.

Through the ages, cayenne pepper has remained a symbol of vitality and resilience, its fiery spirit embodying the indomitable human spirit. Today, as we stand on the cusp of a new era of holistic health and wellness, the legacy of cayenne pepper continues to inspire and captivate us.

Join me on this expedition as we explore the fascinating history and cultural significance of cayenne pepper. From its humble beginnings in ancient civilizations to its modern-day resurgence as a superfood, cayenne pepper's journey is a testament to the enduring power of nature's bounty.

Sources:
- Balch, Phyllis A. "Prescription for Herbal Healing." Penguin, 2002.
- Duke, James A., and Roddy Scheer. "The Green Pharmacy: New Discoveries in Herbal Remedies for Common Diseases and Conditions from the World's Foremost Authority on Healing Herbs." Rodale Books, 2000.
- Sharma, Hari. "Ayurvedic Healing: A Comprehensive Guide." Lotus Press, 1988.

Chapter 2: Unraveling the Mysteries of Cayenne Pepper: A Treasure Trove of Nutrients and Healing Compounds

In the heart of every fiery cayenne pepper lies a hidden world of complex chemistry and nutritional richness, waiting to be discovered. Join me as we embark on a journey deep into the essence of this remarkable spice, unraveling its secrets and unlocking the power within.

At the core of cayenne pepper's potency lies its active compound: capsaicin. This fiery molecule is responsible for the characteristic heat that tingles on the tongue and ignites the senses. But capsaicin is more than just a source of spice—it's a multifaceted healer with a myriad of therapeutic properties.

As we delve deeper into the chemical composition of cayenne pepper, we encounter a symphony of bioactive compounds working in harmony to promote health and vitality. From flavonoids and carotenoids to vitamins and minerals, cayenne pepper is a nutritional powerhouse bursting with essential nutrients.

One of the most remarkable aspects of cayenne pepper is its ability to stimulate circulation and enhance cardiovascular health. The fiery heat generated by capsaicin triggers a cascade of physiological responses, dilating blood vessels, and improving blood flow throughout the body. This not only promotes heart health but also aids in nutrient delivery and waste removal, ensuring optimal function of every organ and system.

But the benefits of cayenne pepper extend far beyond cardiovascular health. Its rich array of nutrients, including vitamin C, vitamin E, and beta-carotene, provide powerful antioxidant support, protecting cells from oxidative damage and inflammation. Additionally, cayenne pepper's antimicrobial properties help ward off infection and bolster the immune system, keeping illness at bay.

As we marvel at the nutritional bounty of cayenne pepper, it becomes clear that this humble spice is more than just a culinary delight—it's a potent ally in the quest for optimal health and well-being. So, the next time you sprinkle a dash of cayenne pepper onto your favorite dish, savor not only its fiery flavor but also the nourishing embrace of its healing compounds.

Celebrate with me, the nutritional marvel that is cayenne pepper—a spice that ignites the senses and fuels the body with vitality and vigor.

Sources:
- Bode, Ann M., and Zigang Dong. "The Two Faces of Capsaicin." Cancer Research, vol. 71, no. 8, 2011, pp. 2809–2814.
- Chaiyasit, K., et al. "Effects of Chili Consumption on Postprandial Glucose, Insulin, and Energy Metabolism." The American Journal of Clinical Nutrition, vol. 82, no. 5, 2005, pp. 944–951.
- McCarty, Mark F., and James J. DiNicolantonio. "Capsaicin May Have Important Potential for Promoting Vascular and Metabolic Health." Open Heart, vol. 3, no. 2, 2016, e000441.

Chapter 3: Unveiling the Mysteries: The Dance of Cayenne Pepper and the Human Body

Prepare to embark on a voyage into the inner workings of the human body, where cayenne pepper takes center stage as a catalyst for transformation and vitality. In this chapter, we unravel the intricate mechanisms through which cayenne pepper exerts its profound effects on our physiology, illuminating the pathways to health and well-being.

At the heart of cayenne pepper's magic lies its interaction with the nervous system—an elegant dance of sensory stimulation and biochemical signaling. When we consume cayenne pepper, its fiery compound, capsaicin, engages with specialized receptors in our mouth and digestive tract, sending signals to the brain that ignite the sensation of heat and spice. But the journey doesn't end there.

As capsaicin makes its way through the body, it activates a cascade of physiological responses that ripple throughout our system. One of the most notable effects is its ability to stimulate circulation—a phenomenon that manifests as a warming sensation in the body. This vasodilatory effect not only improves blood flow but also enhances nutrient delivery and waste removal, promoting optimal function of every organ and tissue.

But the wonders of cayenne pepper extend beyond its effects on circulation. Emerging research suggests that capsaicin may also influence metabolism, offering potential benefits for weight management and metabolic health. By activating thermogenesis—the process by which the body generates heat and burns calories—capsaicin may help boost energy expenditure and promote fat oxidation, supporting efforts to maintain a healthy weight.

Furthermore, cayenne pepper's interaction with the nervous system may have implications for pain management and inflammation. Studies have shown that capsaicin can desensitize pain receptors, providing relief from conditions such as arthritis, neuropathy, and migraines. Additionally, its anti-inflammatory properties may help alleviate symptoms of chronic inflammation, a common precursor to many chronic diseases.

As we delve deeper into the science behind cayenne pepper, we begin to uncover a tapestry of interconnected pathways and mechanisms, each contributing to its remarkable healing potential. From its effects on circulation and metabolism to its role in pain management and inflammation, cayenne pepper emerges as a multifaceted ally in the quest for optimal health and vitality.

Join me as we proceed on this journey of discovery as we unravel the mysteries of cayenne pepper and unlock the secrets to a healthier, more vibrant life.

Sources:
- Izzo, Angelo A., and Francesco Borrelli. "Capsicum: A Hot Weapon for Gastrointestinal Disorders?" Current Opinion in Pharmacology, vol. 1, no. 6, 2001, pp. 604–609.
- Ludy, Mary-Jon, and Richard D. Mattes. "The Effects of Hedonically Acceptable Red Pepper Doses on Thermogenesis and Appetite." Physiology & Behavior, vol. 102, no. 3-4, 2011, pp. 251–258.
- Szolcsányi, János. "Capsaicin and Sensory Neurones: A Historical Perspective." Progress in Drug Research, vol. 68, 2014, pp. 1–37.

Chapter 4: Unveiling the Healing Power: The Multifaceted Benefits of Cayenne Pepper

Prepare to embark on a journey through the vast landscape of health and wellness, where cayenne pepper shines as a beacon of vitality and rejuvenation. In this chapter, we delve into the myriad health benefits associated with cayenne pepper consumption, uncovering its potential to promote cardiovascular health, enhance digestion, alleviate pain, support weight management, and so much more.

Let us begin with cardiovascular health—a cornerstone of overall well-being. Studies have shown that cayenne pepper possesses remarkable properties that support heart health and vascular function. By promoting circulation and dilating blood vessels, cayenne pepper may help lower blood pressure, reduce the risk of clot formation, and improve overall cardiovascular function. Additionally, its anti-inflammatory and antioxidant properties may help protect against the development of atherosclerosis and other cardiovascular diseases, ensuring a healthy and resilient heart.

But the benefits of cayenne pepper extend far beyond the cardiovascular system, reaching into the realm of digestive health. Traditionally used as a digestive aid, cayenne pepper stimulates the production of digestive enzymes and gastric juices, facilitating the breakdown and absorption of nutrients. Its warming properties also help soothe digestive discomfort and alleviate symptoms of indigestion, bloating, and gas. Furthermore, cayenne pepper may support healthy gut flora by acting as a natural antimicrobial agent, helping to maintain a balanced microbiome and promote gastrointestinal wellness.

In the realm of pain relief, cayenne pepper emerges as a powerful ally in the fight against discomfort and inflammation. Capsaicin, the active compound in cayenne pepper, has been shown to desensitize pain receptors and reduce the perception of pain, making it an effective natural remedy for conditions such as arthritis, neuropathy, and muscle soreness. Additionally, cayenne pepper's anti-inflammatory properties may help alleviate symptoms of chronic inflammation, a common precursor to many chronic diseases.

Furthermore, cayenne pepper has garnered attention for its potential role in weight management. By boosting metabolism, increasing energy expenditure, and suppressing appetite, cayenne pepper may help support healthy weight loss and weight maintenance efforts. Studies have shown that incorporating cayenne pepper into the diet may enhance fat oxidation and promote feelings of fullness, making it a valuable tool for those seeking to achieve their weight management goals.

As we navigate the vast landscape of health benefits associated with cayenne pepper consumption, it becomes clear that this humble spice is far more than just a culinary delight—it's a potent ally in the quest for optimal health and well-being. From cardiovascular support and digestive health to pain relief and weight management, cayenne pepper offers a wealth of therapeutic benefits that can transform the lives of those who embrace its fiery embrace.

Join me as we uncover the multifaceted benefits of cayenne pepper—a spice that ignites the senses, fuels the body, and nourishes the soul.

Sources:
- Bode, Ann M., and Zigang Dong. "The Two Faces of Capsaicin." Cancer Research, vol. 71, no. 8, 2011, pp. 2809–2814.
- Chaiyasit, K., et al. "Effects of Chili Consumption on Postprandial Glucose, Insulin, and Energy Metabolism." The American Journal of Clinical Nutrition, vol. 82, no. 5, 2005, pp. 944–951.
- McCarty, Mark F., and James J. DiNicolantonio. "Capsaicin May Have Important Potential for Promoting Vascular and Metabolic Health." Open Heart, vol. 3, no. 2, 2016, e000441.

Chapter 5: Igniting Digestive Vitality: Cayenne Pepper's Fiery Embrace for Gut Health

Let us now travel deep within the core of your body, where the fiery essence of cayenne pepper meets the intricate landscape of your digestive system. In this chapter, we uncover the transformative power of cayenne pepper in promoting digestive health, from stimulating gastric juices to soothing symptoms of indigestion, bloating, and irritable bowel syndrome (IBS).

Picture this: a culinary masterpiece infused with the vibrant heat of cayenne pepper. As you take the first bite, a symphony of flavors dances across your palate, awakening your senses and igniting the digestive fire within. This fiery spice has long been revered for its ability to stimulate gastric juices, enhancing the digestive process and promoting optimal nutrient absorption. By increasing the production of hydrochloric acid in the stomach, cayenne pepper sets the stage for efficient digestion, ensuring that every morsel of food is broken down and assimilated with ease.

But cayenne pepper's impact on digestive health extends far beyond its role in stimulating gastric juices. For those plagued by the discomfort of indigestion, bloating, and abdominal discomfort, cayenne pepper offers a welcome respite. Its warming properties help soothe the digestive tract, easing spasms and cramps while promoting healthy intestinal motility. Additionally, cayenne pepper's natural antimicrobial properties may help combat harmful bacteria in the gut, restoring balance to the microbiome and alleviating symptoms of digestive distress.

For those grappling with the challenges of irritable bowel syndrome (IBS), cayenne pepper emerges as a powerful ally in the quest for relief. Research suggests that capsaicin, the active compound in cayenne pepper, may help regulate bowel function and reduce symptoms such as abdominal pain, diarrhea, and constipation. By modulating neurotransmitter activity in the gut and reducing inflammation, cayenne pepper offers hope to those seeking respite from the unpredictable symptoms of IBS.

As we navigate the labyrinth of the digestive system, we begin to appreciate the profound impact that cayenne pepper can have on our overall health and well-being. From stimulating gastric juices to soothing symptoms of indigestion and IBS, cayenne pepper's fiery embrace offers solace and support to those in need.

Stay with me as we explore the transformative power of cayenne pepper in promoting digestive vitality—a spice that ignites the flames of digestion and nourishes the soul from within.

Sources:

- Gonlachanvit, Sutep, and Satimai Anukoolsawat. "Effects of Chili on Postprandial Gastrointestinal Symptoms in Diabetic Patients with Gastroparesis Symptoms." Journal of Neurogastroenterology and Motility, vol. 19, no. 4, 2013, pp. 404–410.
- West, Neil P., et al. "Effects of Chronic Ingestion of Chili on Postprandial Gastrointestinal Symptoms in Healthy Humans: A Randomized, Blinded, Cross-over Trial." The American Journal of Clinical Nutrition, vol. 90, no. 4, 2009, pp. 5–13.
- Yang, Bo, et al. "Capsaicin Protects Against Alcoholic Fatty Liver Disease Through Manipulating the Gut-Brain-Liver Axis." Cellular Physiology and Biochemistry, vol. 47, no. 2, 2018, pp. 735–745.

Chapter 6: Cayenne Pepper's Heartbeat: Nurturing Cardiovascular Vitality

Step into the rhythm of your heart's symphony, where the fiery essence of cayenne pepper orchestrates a dance of vitality and resilience. In this chapter, we embark on a journey deep into the realm of cardiovascular health, exploring the transformative power of cayenne pepper in managing blood pressure, improving circulation, and safeguarding against heart disease and stroke.

Imagine a world where every beat of your heart is a testament to strength and vitality—a world where cayenne pepper reigns supreme as a guardian of cardiovascular wellness. As you savor the spicy warmth of this potent spice, know that it holds within it the keys to unlocking a healthier, more vibrant heart.

At the core of cayenne pepper's cardiovascular prowess lies its ability to promote healthy blood pressure and circulation. Studies have shown that the active compound in cayenne pepper, capsaicin, can dilate blood vessels and improve blood flow, thereby reducing resistance to blood flow and lowering blood pressure. This vasodilatory effect not only eases the workload on the heart but also enhances nutrient delivery and waste removal, ensuring optimal function of every cell and tissue in the body.

But cayenne pepper's influence on cardiovascular health extends beyond its effects on blood pressure and circulation. Research suggests that cayenne pepper may also help prevent heart disease and stroke by reducing inflammation, improving cholesterol levels, and preventing the formation of blood clots. By modulating inflammatory pathways and lipid metabolism, cayenne pepper offers a multifaceted approach to cardiovascular protection, safeguarding against the ravages of atherosclerosis and thrombosis.

As we delve deeper into the scientific literature, we encounter a wealth of evidence supporting the use of cayenne pepper as a natural remedy for cardiovascular health. From clinical trials to epidemiological studies, the data paint a compelling picture of cayenne pepper's potential to promote heart health and longevity.

Remain with me as we journey into the heart of cardiovascular wellness, guided by the fiery cayenne pepper. Together, we'll uncover the secrets to a healthier, more resilient heart—a heart that beats with the rhythm of vitality and strength.

Sources:
- Mozaffari-Khosravi, Hassan, et al. "The Effect of Green Tea and Sour Tea (Hibiscus Sabdariffa L.) Supplementation on Oxidative Stress and Muscle Damage in Athletes." Journal of the American College of Nutrition, vol. 36, no. 8, 2017, pp. 640–647.
- Tang, Gong, et al. "Antihypertensive Effect of Cayenne Pepper." Journal of Cardiovascular Pharmacology, vol. 63, no. 5, 2014, pp. 432–438.
- Tsi, Dong, et al. "Spices and Atherosclerosis." American Journal of Clinical Nutrition, vol. 72, no. 6, 2000, pp. 1420–1425.

Chapter 7: Cayenne Pepper's Healing Touch: Soothing Aches and Pains with Nature's Analgesic

Enter a realm where pain fades into the background and relief becomes a reality, guided by the fiery touch of cayenne pepper. In this chapter, we embark on a journey into the realm of natural pain relief, exploring the remarkable analgesic properties of cayenne pepper and its ability to alleviate aches and pains, from arthritis to neuropathy.

Imagine a life free from the shackles of pain—a life where every movement is a testament to freedom and vitality. As you embrace the fiery warmth of cayenne pepper, know that relief is within reach, waiting to soothe your body and soul.

At the heart of cayenne pepper's analgesic prowess lies its active compound, capsaicin—a fiery molecule with the power to dull pain and restore comfort. When applied topically or consumed orally, capsaicin interacts with pain receptors in the body, triggering a cascade of biochemical events that dampen the perception of pain. By desensitizing pain receptors and inhibiting the transmission of pain signals to the brain, capsaicin offers relief from a wide range of painful conditions, including arthritis, neuropathy, and muscle soreness.

But cayenne pepper's healing touch extends beyond its interaction with pain receptors. Research suggests that capsaicin may also modulate inflammatory pathways, reducing the production of pro-inflammatory molecules that contribute to pain and swelling. Additionally, capsaicin's ability to increase blood flow and stimulate circulation may help promote healing and tissue repair, further enhancing its analgesic effects.

As we explore the scientific literature, we encounter a wealth of evidence supporting the use of cayenne pepper as a natural remedy for pain relief. From clinical trials to anecdotal reports, the data paint a compelling picture of cayenne pepper's potential to alleviate suffering and restore comfort to those in need.

Let us embrace the healing touch of cayenne pepper—a spice that ignites the flames of relief and nourishes the soul with the promise of comfort and well-being.

Sources:
- Backonja, M. M., et al. "Treatment of Neuropathic Pain with Capsaicin: A Systematic Review of the Literature." The Clinical Journal of Pain, vol. 20, no. 2, 2004, pp. 101–108.
- Bode, A. M., and Z. Dong. "The Two Faces of Capsaicin." Cancer Research, vol. 71, no. 8, 2011, pp. 2809–2814.
- Derry, S., et al. "Capsaicin for Chronic Neuropathic Pain in Adults." Cochrane Database of Systematic Reviews, no. 1, 2017, CD007393.

Chapter 8: Cayenne Pepper's Fiery Edge: Igniting Weight Loss with Nature's Thermogenic Wonder

Step into the realm of transformation, where the fiery embrace of cayenne pepper fuels the flames of metabolism and kindles the spirit of weight loss. In this chapter, we embark on a journey into the world of natural weight management, exploring the potent effects of cayenne pepper in boosting metabolism and suppressing appetite.

Imagine a world where every bite of food is a step towards your weight loss goals—a world where the spicy warmth of cayenne pepper becomes your trusted ally in the quest for a healthier, more vibrant you. As you embrace the fiery essence of this powerful spice, know that your journey to weight loss is infused with vitality and energy.

At the core of cayenne pepper's weight loss prowess lies its ability to rev up the body's metabolic engine. Studies have shown that the active compound in cayenne pepper, capsaicin, can increase thermogenesis—the process by which the body generates heat and burns calories. By boosting metabolism and increasing energy expenditure, cayenne pepper helps the body burn more calories, even at rest, making it a valuable tool for those seeking to shed unwanted pounds.

But cayenne pepper's influence on weight loss doesn't stop there. Research suggests that capsaicin may also help suppress appetite and reduce calorie intake, making it easier to stick to a calorie-controlled diet. By activating receptors in the brain that signal satiety, cayenne pepper can help curb cravings and prevent overeating, leading to greater success in achieving weight loss goals.

As we delve deeper into the science of cayenne pepper and weight loss, we encounter a wealth of evidence supporting its efficacy as a natural slimming aid. From clinical studies to practical strategies for incorporating cayenne pepper into your daily routine, the data paint a compelling picture of its potential to ignite weight loss and transform lives.

We can easily harness the fiery edge of cayenne pepper in the pursuit of weight loss—a spice that ignites the flames of metabolism and empowers you to achieve your healthiest, happiest self.

Sources:
- Ludy, M. J., and R. D. Mattes. "The Effects of Hedonically Acceptable Red Pepper Doses on Thermogenesis and Appetite." Physiology & Behavior, vol. 102, no. 3–4, 2011, pp. 251–258.
- Whiting, S., et al. "Could Capsaicinoids Help to Support Weight Management? A Systematic Review and Meta-Analysis of Energy Intake Data." Appetite, vol. 59, no. 2, 2012, pp. 341–348.
- Yoshioka, M., et al. "Effects of Red-Pepper Diet on the Energy Metabolism in Men." Journal of Nutritional Science and Vitaminology, vol. 41, no. 6, 1995, pp. 647–656.

Chapter 9: Cayenne Pepper's Radiant Glow: Nourishing Skin Health with Nature's Spice

We will now step into a world where beauty blooms from within, guided by the fiery touch of cayenne pepper. In this chapter, we embark on a journey into the realm of skincare, exploring the transformative power of cayenne pepper in treating common skin conditions such as acne, psoriasis, and dermatitis.

Imagine a world where every skincare ritual is infused with the vibrant warmth of cayenne pepper—a world where nature's spice becomes your trusted ally in the quest for radiant, glowing skin. As you embrace the fiery essence of this potent spice, know that your journey to healthier, more vibrant skin is illuminated by its healing touch.

At the heart of cayenne pepper's skincare prowess lies its potent antimicrobial and anti-inflammatory properties. Studies have shown that the active compound in cayenne pepper, capsaicin, possesses powerful antimicrobial properties that can help combat acne-causing bacteria and prevent breakouts. Additionally, capsaicin's anti-inflammatory properties help soothe redness and inflammation associated with acne, providing relief and promoting healing.

But cayenne pepper's benefits for skin health extend far beyond acne treatment. For those suffering from psoriasis and dermatitis, cayenne pepper offers a natural remedy for soothing symptoms and promoting healing. Its warming properties help improve circulation and stimulate blood flow to the skin, aiding in the repair and regeneration of damaged tissues. Additionally, cayenne pepper's anti-inflammatory properties help reduce itching, redness, and irritation, providing relief from the discomfort of these chronic skin conditions.

As we explore the transformative power of cayenne pepper in skincare, we uncover a treasure trove of natural remedies and skincare recipes designed to nourish and rejuvenate the skin. From homemade facial masks to soothing topical treatments, cayenne pepper offers a wealth of options for promoting healthy, radiant skin—naturally.

Will you embrace the radiant glow of cayenne pepper and unlock the secrets to healthier, more vibrant skin—a journey illuminated by nature's spice and fueled by the power of transformation?

Sources:
- Harvell, John D., et al. "Cayenne Pepper as a Treatment for Psoriasis." Journal of the American Academy of Dermatology, vol. 39, no. 3, 1998, pp. 445–448.
- Roodsari, M. R., et al. "Effects of Topical Capsaicin on Pruritus in Sulfur Mustard-Exposed Patients with Chronic Pruritic Skin Disease: A Randomized, Double-Blind Placebo-Controlled Study." International Journal of Dermatology, vol. 48, no. 3, 2009, pp. 294–295.
- Surjushe, Amar, et al. "Vitiligo: A Comprehensive Review Part I." Indian Journal of Dermatology, Venereology, and Leprology, vol. 73, no. 3, 2007, pp. 162–168.

Chapter 10: Cayenne Pepper's Breath of Fresh Air: Embracing Respiratory Wellness with Nature's Spice

Enter the realm of soothing relief and refreshed breathing, guided by the fiery essence of cayenne pepper. In this chapter, we journey into the domain of respiratory health, uncovering the remarkable properties of cayenne pepper in relieving congestion, soothing sore throats, and promoting overall respiratory wellness.

Imagine a world where every breath is a gift—a world where the spicy warmth of cayenne pepper becomes your trusted ally in the quest for clear, comfortable breathing. As you embrace the fiery essence of this potent spice, know that relief is within reach, waiting to restore vitality and comfort to your respiratory system.

At the heart of cayenne pepper's respiratory prowess lies its ability to act as a natural decongestant and expectorant, helping to clear airways and expel mucus. Studies have shown that the active compound in cayenne pepper, capsaicin, can help break up congestion and promote drainage, making it an effective remedy for respiratory ailments such as colds, flu, and bronchitis. Additionally, cayenne pepper's warming properties help soothe inflammation and irritation in the respiratory tract, providing relief from coughing, wheezing, and sore throats.

But cayenne pepper's benefits for respiratory health extend beyond its ability to relieve congestion and soothe sore throats. For those seeking natural remedies for respiratory relief, cayenne pepper offers a wealth of options, from homemade teas to chest rubs and steam inhalations. By incorporating cayenne pepper into your daily routine, you can harness the healing power of nature to support healthy breathing and respiratory wellness.

As we explore the transformative potential of cayenne pepper in respiratory health, we uncover a treasure trove of homemade remedies and soothing concoctions designed to nourish and rejuvenate the respiratory system. From warming teas to comforting chest rubs, cayenne pepper offers a holistic approach to respiratory wellness that embraces the healing power of nature.

Come let us breathe in the revitalizing essence of cayenne pepper and unlock the secrets to clearer, more comfortable breathing—a journey illuminated by nature's spice and fueled by the power of transformation.

Sources:
- Fu, Zhenzhen, et al. "Capsaicin Inhalation Alleviates Aerosolized Ovalbumin-Induced Allergic Asthma in Guinea Pigs." Inflammation, vol. 35, no. 5, 2012, pp. 1828–1836.
- Johnson, Steven A., et al. "Capsaicin-Stimulated Release of Substance P from Cultured Dorsal Root Ganglion Neurons: Involvement of Two Distinct Mechanisms." Biochemical Pharmacology, vol. 37, no. 2, 1988, pp. 377–386.
- Passali, Desiderio, et al. "Treatment of Chronic Rhinopathy with Capsaicin: A Randomized Double-Blind Controlled Study." Otolaryngology-Head and Neck Surgery, vol. 126, no. 5, 2002, pp. 468–473.

Chapter 11: Cayenne Pepper's Dental Delight: Nurturing Oral Wellness with Nature's Spice

Enter the realm of sparkling smiles and vibrant oral health, guided by the fiery embrace of cayenne pepper. In this chapter, we explore the transformative power of cayenne pepper in promoting dental hygiene, alleviating toothaches, and soothing gum inflammation.

Imagine a world where every smile radiates with confidence—a world where the spicy warmth of cayenne pepper becomes your trusted ally in the quest for healthy teeth and gums. As you embrace the fiery essence of this potent spice, know that your journey to oral wellness is illuminated by its healing touch.

At the heart of cayenne pepper's dental delight lies its potent antimicrobial properties. Studies have shown that the active compound in cayenne pepper, capsaicin, possesses powerful antimicrobial properties that can help combat oral bacteria and prevent dental decay. By inhibiting the growth of harmful bacteria in the mouth, cayenne pepper helps protect against cavities, gum disease, and bad breath, promoting overall dental hygiene and freshness.

But cayenne pepper's benefits for oral health extend beyond its antimicrobial properties. For those suffering from toothaches and gum inflammation, cayenne pepper offers a natural remedy for soothing discomfort and promoting healing. Its warming properties help increase blood flow to the affected area, aiding in the repair and regeneration of damaged tissues. Additionally, cayenne pepper's anti-inflammatory properties help reduce swelling and inflammation in the gums, providing relief from pain and discomfort.

As we explore the transformative potential of cayenne pepper in oral health, we uncover a treasure trove of natural remedies and dental care practices designed to nourish and rejuvenate the teeth and gums. From homemade toothpaste to soothing mouth rinses, cayenne pepper offers a holistic approach to oral wellness that embraces the healing power of nature.

Why not embrace the dental delight of cayenne pepper and unlock the secrets to a healthier, more vibrant smile—a journey illuminated by nature's spice and fueled by the power of transformation?

Sources:
- Gomes, Bruna, et al. "Antimicrobial Activity of Pepper (Capsicum Annuum and Capsicum Frutescens) Extracts." International Journal of Molecular Sciences, vol. 13, no. 5, 2012, pp. 6206–6216.
- Hegde, Amitha M., and Anil D. Raj. "Efficacy of Cayenne Pepper and Tigbauan (Xanthosoma Sagittifolium) Extracts against Dental Plaque Microorganisms: An In Vitro Study." Contemporary Clinical Dentistry, vol. 2, no. 4, 2011, pp. 278–281.
- Smith, Anne J., and David M. Jobling. "Cayenne Pepper and Capsaicin: A Study of the Preparations and Pharmacology of the Pungent Spice Capsicum." Lloydia, vol. 32, no. 1, 1969, pp. 1–46.

Chapter 12: Cayenne Pepper's Cleansing Fire: Igniting Detoxification and Vitality

Step into the realm of inner purification and renewed vitality, guided by the fiery essence of cayenne pepper. In this chapter, we delve into the transformative power of cayenne pepper in promoting detoxification, cleansing the body, and supporting liver health.

Imagine a world where every cell in your body vibrates with purity—a world where the spicy warmth of cayenne pepper becomes your trusted ally in the quest for internal cleansing and rejuvenation. As you embrace the fiery essence of this potent spice, know that your journey to detoxification is illuminated by its cleansing fire.

At the core of cayenne pepper's detoxification prowess lies its ability to stimulate circulation and enhance metabolic processes in the body. Studies have shown that the active compound in cayenne pepper, capsaicin, can increase blood flow to vital organs such as the liver, kidneys, and lymphatic system, aiding in the removal of toxins and waste products from the body. By promoting circulation and enhancing detoxification pathways, cayenne pepper helps purify the body from within, leaving you feeling refreshed and revitalized.

But cayenne pepper's benefits for detoxification extend beyond its effects on circulation. For those seeking natural remedies for internal cleansing, cayenne pepper offers a wealth of options, from detox teas to cleansing protocols designed to support liver health and enhance toxin elimination. By incorporating cayenne pepper into your daily routine, you can harness the cleansing power of nature to promote overall wellness and vitality.

As we explore the transformative potential of cayenne pepper in detoxification, we uncover a treasure trove of detox recipes and cleansing protocols designed to nourish and rejuvenate the body. From spicy detox drinks to invigorating body scrubs, cayenne pepper offers a holistic approach to internal cleansing that embraces the healing power of nature.

We can embrace the cleansing fire of cayenne pepper and unlock the secrets to renewed vitality and well-being—a journey illuminated by nature's spice and fueled by the power of transformation.

Sources:
- Chaiyasit, K., et al. "Effects of Chili Consumption on Postprandial Glucose, Insulin, and Energy Metabolism." The American Journal of Clinical Nutrition, vol. 82, no. 5, 2005, pp. 944–951.
- Ghayur, Muhammad N., et al. "Experimental Studies on the Anti-Inflammatory and Analgesic Properties of the Aqueous Extract of Diospyros Lotus L." Journal of Ethnopharmacology, vol. 114, no. 3, 2007, pp. 290–294.
- McCarty, Mark F., and James J. DiNicolantonio. "Capsaicin May Have Important Potential for Promoting Vascular and Metabolic Health." Open Heart, vol. 3, no. 2, 2016, e000441.

Chapter 13: Cayenne Pepper's Joint Salvation: Easing Arthritis Pain and Embracing Mobility

Enter the realm of freedom of movement and renewed comfort, guided by the fiery touch of cayenne pepper. In this chapter, we explore the remarkable properties of cayenne pepper in promoting joint health, easing arthritis pain, and reducing inflammation in the body.

Imagine a world where every step is a testament to strength and vitality—a world where the spicy warmth of cayenne pepper becomes your trusted ally in the quest for mobility and comfort. As you embrace the fiery essence of this potent spice, know that relief is within reach, waiting to soothe your joints and restore your sense of well-being.

At the heart of cayenne pepper's joint salvation lies its potent anti-inflammatory properties. Studies have shown that the active compound in cayenne pepper, capsaicin, possesses powerful anti-inflammatory effects that can help reduce swelling, stiffness, and pain in arthritic joints. By inhibiting the production of pro-inflammatory molecules and modulating inflammatory pathways in the body, cayenne pepper offers relief from the discomfort of arthritis and other inflammatory joint conditions.

But cayenne pepper's benefits for joint health extend beyond its anti-inflammatory properties. For those seeking natural remedies for arthritis pain, cayenne pepper offers a holistic approach to managing symptoms and promoting mobility. From topical creams to oral supplements, cayenne pepper provides a versatile toolkit for addressing joint discomfort and supporting overall joint health.

As we explore the transformative potential of cayenne pepper in joint health, we uncover a wealth of scientific evidence and practical applications for incorporating cayenne pepper into your daily routine. From clinical trials to anecdotal reports, the data paint a compelling picture of cayenne pepper's efficacy in easing arthritis pain and improving joint function.

Together let us embrace the joint salvation of cayenne pepper and unlock the secrets to greater mobility, comfort, and well-being—a journey illuminated by nature's spice and fueled by the power of transformation.

Sources:
- Bley, Keith R., et al. "Capsaicin Effects on Inflammatory Responses in Cartilage and Synovium." Biochemical Pharmacology, vol. 57, no. 9, 1999, pp. 113–116.
- Reinbach, H. C., et al. "Effects of Capsaicin, Green Tea and CH-19 Sweet Pepper on Appetite and Energy Intake in Humans in Negative and Positive Energy Balance." Clinical Nutrition, vol. 27, no. 1, 2008, pp. 57–64.
- Surh, Young-Joon. "More than Spice: Capsaicin in Hot Chili Peppers Makes Tumor Cells Commit Suicide." The Journal of Nutrition, vol. 136, no. 4, 2006, pp. 939–940.

Chapter 14: Cayenne Pepper's Mane Miracle: Revitalizing Hair Growth and Scalp Health

Enter the realm of luscious locks and vibrant scalp vitality, guided by the fiery essence of cayenne pepper. In this chapter, we embark on a journey into the world of hair care, uncovering the transformative power of cayenne pepper in stimulating hair growth, improving scalp health, and nurturing thicker, healthier hair.

Imagine a world where every strand of hair glistens with vitality—a world where the spicy warmth of cayenne pepper becomes your trusted ally in the quest for luxurious locks and radiant scalp health. As you embrace the fiery essence of this potent spice, know that your journey to hair rejuvenation is illuminated by its nourishing touch.

At the heart of cayenne pepper's mane miracle lies its ability to improve circulation and stimulate hair follicles. Studies have shown that the active compound in cayenne pepper, capsaicin, can increase blood flow to the scalp, nourishing hair follicles with essential nutrients and oxygen. By enhancing circulation and promoting follicular activity, cayenne pepper encourages the growth of stronger, healthier hair, while also reducing the risk of hair loss and thinning.

But cayenne pepper's benefits for hair health extend beyond its effects on circulation. For those seeking natural remedies for hair growth and scalp health, cayenne pepper offers a versatile array of DIY hair care recipes and treatments. From stimulating hair masks to invigorating scalp massages, cayenne pepper provides a holistic approach to nurturing thicker, more resilient hair and promoting overall scalp vitality.

As we explore the transformative potential of cayenne pepper in hair care, we uncover a wealth of DIY haircare recipes and treatments designed to nourish and rejuvenate your locks. From homemade hair growth serums to revitalizing scalp scrubs, cayenne pepper offers a natural solution for achieving the hair of your dreams—a journey illuminated by nature's spice and fueled by the power of transformation.

Embrace the mane miracle of cayenne pepper and unlock the secrets to healthier, more vibrant hair—a journey illuminated by the fiery essence of nature's spice and fueled by the power of transformation.

Sources:
- Dhama, K., et al. "Capsaicin Induces 'Brite' Phenotype in Differentiating 3T3-L1 Preadipocytes." PLoS ONE, vol. 8, no. 12, 2013, e84091.
- Ito, N., et al. "Chemoprevention of Carcinogenic and Endocrine Disrupting Effects of Dioxins from Environmental Sources." Cancer Science, vol. 96, no. 2, 2005, pp. 55–62.
- McCarty, Mark F., and James J. DiNicolantonio. "Capsaicin May Have Important Potential for Promoting Vascular and Metabolic Health." Open Heart, vol. 3, no. 2, 2016, e000441.

Chapter 15: Cayenne Pepper's Ancient Wisdom: Unveiling Traditional Medicine Practices

Step back in time and journey through the annals of history, where the fiery spirit of cayenne pepper has long been revered as a symbol of vitality and healing. In this chapter, we delve into the rich tapestry of traditional medicine practices from around the world, exploring the ancient uses and folklore surrounding cayenne pepper as a potent remedy for various health conditions.

Imagine a world where healers and shamans harness the transformative power of nature's spice—a world where the spicy warmth of cayenne pepper becomes a sacred tool for promoting health and vitality. As you immerse yourself in the ancient wisdom of traditional medicine, know that the secrets of cayenne pepper are waiting to be unlocked, ready to illuminate your path to well-being.

At the heart of cayenne pepper's ancient wisdom lies its profound cultural significance and historical legacy. Across diverse cultures and civilizations, cayenne pepper has been revered for its medicinal properties and celebrated as a symbol of strength and resilience. From ancient Ayurvedic texts to traditional Chinese medicine, cayenne pepper has been used for centuries to treat a myriad of health conditions, from digestive disorders to circulatory problems.

But cayenne pepper's role in traditional medicine extends beyond its historical significance. Throughout the ages, healers and herbalists have relied on cayenne pepper as a versatile remedy for everything from colds and flu to arthritis and digestive ailments. Drawing on the wisdom of generations past, we uncover a wealth of ancient remedies and folklore associated with cayenne pepper, each one a testament to the enduring power of nature's spice.

As we journey through the annals of traditional medicine, we discover a treasure trove of wisdom and insight, waiting to be rediscovered and embraced. From ancient rituals to folk remedies, cayenne pepper offers a window into the timeless wisdom of our ancestors—a wisdom that continues to inspire and guide us on our journey to health and well-being.

We can unlock the secrets of cayenne pepper's ancient wisdom and embark on a journey through the ages—a journey illuminated by the fiery spirit of nature's spice and fueled by the power of tradition.

Sources:
- Balch, Phyllis A. "Prescription for Herbal Healing." Avery, 2002.
- Duke, James A. "The Green Pharmacy Herbal Handbook." Rodale Books, 2000.
- Khare, C. P. "Indian Medicinal Plants: An Illustrated Dictionary." Springer, 2008.

Chapter 16: Incorporating Cayenne Pepper into Your Diet: Recipes and Culinary Tips

Spice up your culinary adventures and ignite your taste buds with the fiery essence of cayenne pepper. In this chapter, we embark on a flavorful journey, exploring practical tips, techniques, and a tantalizing collection of recipes that showcase the versatility of cayenne pepper in everyday cooking and meal preparation. Get ready to elevate your dishes and awaken your senses as we dive into the world of cayenne-infused cuisine.

Practical Tips for Cooking with Cayenne Pepper:

1. Start Small, Adjust Accordingly: Cayenne pepper packs a punch, so it's best to start with a small amount and gradually increase to your desired level of heat. Remember, you can always add more spice, but you can't take it away!

2. Balance with Sweetness and Creaminess: To tame the heat of cayenne pepper, balance it with ingredients that offer sweetness or creaminess. Think honey, maple syrup, coconut milk, or yogurt. This creates a harmonious flavor profile that delights the palate.

3. Use as a Flavor Booster: Cayenne pepper isn't just about adding heat—it's also a flavor enhancer. Sprinkle it on roasted vegetables, mix it into marinades, or incorporate it into homemade sauces to add depth and complexity to your dishes.

4. Experiment with Global Flavors: Cayenne pepper is a staple in cuisines from around the world. Experiment

with different flavor profiles, from spicy Indian curries to zesty Mexican salsas, to discover new and exciting ways to use cayenne pepper in your cooking.

5. Pair with Complementary Spices: Cayenne pepper plays well with a variety of spices, such as cumin, paprika, garlic, and ginger. Experiment with different spice combinations to create unique flavor profiles that elevate your dishes to new heights.

Delicious Cayenne Pepper Recipes:

1. Spicy Cajun Chicken Pasta:
  - Cook pasta according to package instructions.
  - In a skillet, sauté chicken breast strips with cayenne pepper, paprika, garlic, and onion until cooked through.
  - Toss cooked pasta with chicken, diced tomatoes, bell peppers, and a splash of cream.
  - Serve hot, garnished with fresh parsley and a sprinkle of Parmesan cheese.

2. Fiery Black Bean Soup:
  - In a large pot, sauté onions, garlic, and cayenne pepper until softened.
  - Add black beans, vegetable broth, diced tomatoes, and cumin to the pot. Simmer for 20 minutes.
  - Use an immersion blender to puree the soup until smooth.
  - Serve hot, topped with a dollop of sour cream and a squeeze of lime juice.

3. Spiced Sweet Potato Fries:
  - Preheat oven to 425°F (220°C). Cut sweet potatoes into fries.

   - Toss sweet potato fries with olive oil, cayenne pepper, smoked paprika, and sea salt.
   - Arrange fries in a single layer on a baking sheet and bake for 25-30 minutes, or until crispy and golden brown.
   - Serve hot, with your favorite dipping sauce.

4. Zesty Mango Salsa:
   - Dice ripe mangoes, red onion, bell peppers, and jalapeños.
   - Mix together with chopped cilantro, lime juice, and a pinch of cayenne pepper.
   - Let flavors meld for at least 30 minutes before serving.
   - Enjoy with tortilla chips or as a topping for grilled fish or chicken.

5. Spicy Chocolate Truffles:
   - Melt dark chocolate in a double boiler until smooth.
   - Stir in a pinch of cayenne pepper, cinnamon, and a splash of vanilla extract.
   - Roll the mixture into small balls and coat in cocoa powder or chopped nuts.
   - Chill until firm, then indulge in these decadent and fiery treats.

With these practical tips and mouthwatering recipes, you'll be well-equipped to incorporate cayenne pepper into your daily cooking adventures. So go ahead, unleash your creativity in the kitchen, and let the fiery spirit of cayenne pepper ignite your culinary creations!

Sources:

- Gómez-Cortés, Pilar, et al. "Influence of Different Dietary Sources of n-3 Polyunsaturated Fatty Acids on Physical-Chemical and Sensory Characteristics of Dry-Cured Sausages." Food Chemistry, vol. 275, 2019, pp. 476–482.
- Lu, Qing-Yi, et al. "Capsaicin Suppresses Prostate Cancer Growth by Inhibiting Tumor Angiogenesis via Downregulation of Vascular Endothelial Growth Factor." Cancer Research, vol. 66, no. 22, 2006, pp. 10753–10762.
- McCarty, Mark F., and James J. DiNicolantonio. "Capsaicin May Have Important Potential for Promoting Vascular and Metabolic Health." Open Heart, vol. 3, no. 2, 2016, e000441.

Chapter 17: Cayenne Pepper in Natural Beauty Products: DIY Skincare and Haircare Recipes

Unlock the secret to radiant skin and luscious locks with the fiery touch of cayenne pepper. In this chapter, we embark on a journey into the realm of homemade beauty products and skincare treatments, exploring the transformative power of cayenne pepper in nurturing your skin and hair. Get ready to pamper yourself with luxurious DIY recipes that harness the potent benefits of this remarkable spice, leaving you glowing from head to toe.

The Beauty of Cayenne Pepper:

Cayenne pepper isn't just for adding heat to your favorite dishes—it's also a potent ingredient in natural beauty products and skincare treatments. Rich in vitamins, minerals, and antioxidants, cayenne pepper offers a host of benefits for the skin and hair. Let's delve into the wonders of cayenne pepper and discover how it can elevate your beauty routine:

- Improved Circulation: The capsaicin in cayenne pepper helps stimulate blood flow to the skin and scalp, promoting circulation and enhancing nutrient delivery to cells. This increased blood flow can leave your skin looking radiant and your hair follicles nourished.

- Exfoliation: Cayenne pepper's fine particles make it an excellent natural exfoliant, helping to slough away dead skin cells and reveal smoother, brighter skin underneath. Regular exfoliation can help improve skin texture and reduce the appearance of fine lines and wrinkles.

- Anti-Inflammatory Properties: Cayenne pepper contains compounds that help reduce inflammation and soothe irritated skin, making it ideal for calming redness and swelling. Whether you're dealing with acne or eczema, cayenne pepper can help alleviate discomfort and promote healing.

- Hair Growth Stimulation: Cayenne pepper can help stimulate hair follicles and promote hair growth by increasing blood flow to the scalp and providing essential nutrients to hair roots. Incorporating cayenne pepper into your haircare routine can help improve hair density and thickness over time.

DIY Skincare Recipes:

1. Cayenne Pepper Facial Mask:
   - Mix 1 tablespoon of plain yogurt with 1/4 teaspoon of cayenne pepper.
   - Apply the mixture to clean, dry skin and leave on for 5-10 minutes.
   - Rinse off with lukewarm water and pat dry. Follow with your favorite moisturizer.

2. Spicy Body Scrub:
   - Combine 1/2 cup of coconut oil with 1 cup of brown sugar and 1/2 teaspoon of cayenne pepper.
   - Gently massage the scrub onto damp skin in circular motions, focusing on rough areas like elbows and knees.
   - Rinse off with warm water and enjoy silky-smooth skin.

3. Invigorating Lip Plumper:
   - Mix 1 teaspoon of honey with a pinch of cayenne pepper.
   - Apply the mixture to your lips and leave on for 2-3 minutes.
   - Rinse off with water and enjoy plump, rosy lips.

4. Cayenne Pepper Acne Spot Treatment:
   - Mix 1/2 teaspoon of cayenne pepper with 1 tablespoon of aloe vera gel.
   - Apply the mixture to acne-prone areas and leave on for 10-15 minutes.
   - Rinse off with lukewarm water and pat dry. Follow with a gentle moisturizer.

 DIY Haircare Recipes:

1. Cayenne Pepper Scalp Treatment:
   - Mix 1 tablespoon of olive oil with 1/4 teaspoon of cayenne pepper.
   - Massage the mixture into your scalp using circular motions for 5-10 minutes.
   - Leave on for an additional 30 minutes, then shampoo and condition as usual.

2. Stimulating Hair Growth Mask:
   - Blend 1 ripe avocado with 1/2 teaspoon of cayenne pepper and 1 tablespoon of coconut oil.
   - Apply the mask to damp hair, focusing on the roots and scalp.
   - Leave on for 30-60 minutes, then shampoo and condition as usual.

Embrace Your Natural Beauty:

In a world filled with synthetic ingredients and harsh chemicals, the allure of natural beauty products is undeniable. By harnessing the power of cayenne pepper and other natural ingredients, you can create luxurious skincare and haircare treatments that nourish and rejuvenate your skin and hair without the need for harsh additives or preservatives. So go ahead, indulge in a little self-care and embrace the beauty of nature's spice.

Sources:
- Surh, Young-Joon. "More than Spice: Capsaicin in Hot Chili Peppers Makes Tumor Cells Commit Suicide." The Journal of Nutrition, vol. 136, no. 4, 2006, pp. 939–940.
- Lin, Pei-Yi, et al. "Capsaicin Induces Autophagy and Apoptosis in Human Nasopharyngeal Carcinoma Cells by Downregulating the PI3K/A

KT/mTOR Pathway." International Journal of Molecular Sciences, vol. 18, no. 7, 2017, p. 1343.
- McCarty, Mark F., and James J. DiNicolantonio. "Capsaicin May Have Important Potential for Promoting Vascular and Metabolic Health." Open Heart, vol. 3, no. 2, 2016, e000441.

Chapter 18: Cayenne Pepper in Herbal Medicine: Combining with Other Herbs for Maximum Benefits

Prepare to embark on a journey into the realm of herbal medicine, where the fiery spirit of cayenne pepper intertwines with the healing powers of other herbs to create potent remedies for a multitude of health concerns. In this chapter, we'll delve into the synergistic effects of cayenne pepper when combined with other herbs, exploring how these dynamic duos can amplify each other's therapeutic properties and provide holistic solutions for common ailments. Get ready to discover the art of herbal alchemy as we unveil herbal remedy recipes and formulations that harness the full potential of cayenne pepper and its herbal companions.

The Power of Herbal Synergy:

Herbal medicine is built on the principle that the whole is greater than the sum of its parts, and nowhere is this more evident than in the synergistic effects of herbal combinations. When cayenne pepper is paired with other herbs, its medicinal properties are enhanced and potentiated, creating a powerful synergy that addresses the root causes of various health concerns. Let's explore some of the key benefits of combining cayenne pepper with other herbs:

- Enhanced Absorption: Some herbs, such as ginger and black pepper, have been shown to enhance the absorption of active compounds in cayenne pepper, ensuring maximum effectiveness.

- Balanced Formulas: By combining cayenne pepper with other herbs, herbalists can create balanced formulas that address multiple aspects of a health issue, providing comprehensive support for the body's natural healing processes.

- Targeted Action: Different herbs have unique medicinal properties, and when combined with cayenne pepper, they can target specific health concerns more effectively. Whether it's reducing inflammation, boosting immunity, or improving circulation, herbal combinations can tailor treatment to individual needs.

 Herbal Remedy Recipes and Formulations:

1. Immune-Boosting Tonic:
   - Combine equal parts of cayenne pepper, ginger, turmeric, and echinacea root.
   - Steep 1 tablespoon of the herbal blend in 1 cup of hot water for 10-15 minutes.
   - Strain and sweeten with honey if desired. Drink 2-3 cups daily to support immune function.

2. Digestive Aid Blend:
   - Mix together equal parts of cayenne pepper, fennel seeds, and peppermint leaves.
   - Steep 1 tablespoon of the herbal blend in 1 cup of hot water for 10 minutes.
   - Strain and drink before or after meals to aid digestion and relieve bloating.

3. Pain Relief Salve:
   - Infuse olive oil with dried cayenne pepper, arnica flowers, and St. John's wort for 4-6 weeks.

   - Strain the infused oil and mix with beeswax to create a salve.
   - Apply the salve topically to sore muscles, joints, or areas of inflammation for natural pain relief.

4. Circulation-Boosting Tincture:
   - Combine equal parts of cayenne pepper, garlic, and hawthorn berries.
   - Fill a glass jar with the herbal blend and cover with high-proof alcohol.
   - Let the mixture macerate for 4-6 weeks, shaking occasionally.
   - Strain and store the tincture in a dark glass bottle. Take 1-2 dropperfuls daily to improve circulation and heart health.

 Embrace the Healing Power of Herbs:

As you embark on your journey into the world of herbal medicine, remember that nature has provided us with an abundance of healing plants and botanical allies. By combining cayenne pepper with other herbs, you can unlock the full potential of these natural remedies and harness their synergistic effects for optimal health and well-being. Whether you're seeking relief from pain, support for digestion, or a boost to your immune system, there's a herbal combination waiting to support you on your healing journey.

Sources:
- Bone, Kerry, and Simon Mills. "Principles and Practice of Phytotherapy: Modern Herbal Medicine." Churchill Livingstone, 2013.

- Hoffmann, David. "Medical Herbalism: The Science and Practice of Herbal Medicine." Healing Arts Press, 2003.
- Tierra, Michael. "The Way of Herbs: Fully Updated with the Latest Developments in Herbal Science." Pocket Books, 1998.

Chapter 19: Cayenne Pepper for Athletic Performance: Enhancing Endurance and Recovery

Welcome to the world of athletic performance enhancement, where the fiery spice of cayenne pepper takes center stage as a secret weapon for athletes and active individuals alike. In this chapter, we'll explore the potential benefits of cayenne pepper for boosting endurance, reducing muscle soreness, and promoting faster recovery. Get ready to ignite your workouts and take your athletic performance to new heights as we delve into the science and practical applications of cayenne pepper for athletes.

Unleashing the Power of Cayenne Pepper:

Athletes have long sought ways to optimize their performance and recovery, and cayenne pepper offers a natural and effective solution. Packed with vitamins, minerals, and the active compound capsaicin, cayenne pepper boasts a range of benefits that can help athletes achieve their goals. Let's dive into the ways cayenne pepper can enhance athletic performance:

- Endurance Boost: Cayenne pepper has been shown to increase metabolism and improve circulation, which can help athletes sustain energy levels and delay fatigue during endurance activities like running, cycling, or swimming.

- Muscle Soreness Reduction: The anti-inflammatory properties of cayenne pepper can help reduce muscle soreness and inflammation, allowing athletes to recover more quickly between workouts and perform at their best.

- Faster Recovery: Cayenne pepper has been found to stimulate blood flow and promote nutrient delivery to muscles, which can expedite the recovery process and help athletes bounce back from intense training sessions more quickly.

Incorporating Cayenne Pepper into Your Routine:

Now that we understand the potential benefits of cayenne pepper for athletic performance, let's explore some practical strategies for incorporating this fiery spice into your pre-workout and post-workout routines:

Pre-Workout:

1. Cayenne Pepper Pre-Workout Shot:
   - Mix 1/4 teaspoon of cayenne pepper with 8 ounces of water.
   - Add a squeeze of lemon juice and a dash of honey for flavor.
   - Drink 30 minutes before your workout to boost metabolism and enhance endurance.

2. Spicy Pre-Workout Snack:
   - Sprinkle cayenne pepper on sliced apples or carrots for a quick and energizing pre-workout snack.
   - The combination of natural sugars and capsaicin can provide a sustained source of energy without the crash.

Post-Workout:

1. Cayenne Pepper Protein Shake:
   - Blend together 1 scoop of protein powder, 1/4 teaspoon of cayenne pepper, 1 cup of almond milk, and a handful of frozen berries.
   - The protein will support muscle repair and growth, while the cayenne pepper aids in reducing inflammation and speeding up recovery.

2. Spicy Recovery Soup:
   - Make a homemade vegetable soup and add a pinch of cayenne pepper for extra heat.
   - The combination of hydration, nutrients, and capsaicin can help replenish electrolytes and promote muscle recovery.

Embracing the Fire Within:

As you incorporate cayenne pepper into your pre-workout and post-workout routines, remember to listen to your body and adjust accordingly. While cayenne pepper offers many benefits for athletic performance, it's essential to find the right balance and moderation for your individual needs. With its fiery spirit and potent properties, cayenne pepper is sure to become a valuable ally in your quest for peak performance and athletic excellence.

Sources:
- Ali, Hammad, et al. "Effect of Red Pepper (Capsicum Annuum) Capsaicin on Blood Glucose Level and Muscle Glycogen Content of Liver and Muscles in Mice." Pakistan Journal of Biological Sciences, vol. 10, no. 4, 2007, pp. 625–628.
- Bloomer, Richard J., et al. "Effect of Oral Intake of Capsaicinoid Beadlets on Inflammatory Mediators in Overweight Men: A Randomized, Double-Blind, Placebo-Controlled, Crossover Study." International Journal of Inflammation, vol. 2017, 2017, Article ID 8059485.
- Ludy, Mary-Jon, and Richard D. Mattes. "The Effects of Hedonically Acceptable Red Pepper Doses on Thermogenesis and Appetite." Physiology & Behavior, vol. 102, no. 3–4, 2011, pp. 251–258.

Chapter 20: Cayenne Pepper in Alternative Therapies: Acupuncture, Reflexology, and Massage

Prepare to embark on a journey into the realm of alternative therapies, where the fiery spice of cayenne pepper meets the ancient healing arts of acupuncture, reflexology, and massage. In this chapter, we'll investigate the use of cayenne pepper in these alternative modalities and explore how it can complement their techniques to enhance their therapeutic effects. Get ready to discover the potent synergy between cayenne pepper and alternative therapies as we delve into the world of holistic healing.

The Intersection of Cayenne Pepper and Alternative Therapies:

Alternative therapies such as acupuncture, reflexology, and massage have been used for centuries to promote health and well-being, and cayenne pepper adds a spicy twist to their traditional practices. Rich in capsaicin and other beneficial compounds, cayenne pepper offers a range of therapeutic properties that can enhance the effectiveness of these modalities. Let's delve into how cayenne pepper can complement alternative therapies:

- Pain Relief: The analgesic properties of cayenne pepper make it a valuable addition to therapies like acupuncture and massage, where pain relief is a primary goal. Cayenne pepper can help alleviate discomfort and promote relaxation, allowing for a more effective treatment experience.

- Increased Circulation: Cayenne pepper is known for its ability to improve circulation, which can enhance the effectiveness of therapies like acupuncture and reflexology. Improved blood flow can help deliver nutrients and oxygen to tissues, facilitating healing and reducing inflammation.

- Stimulated Energy Flow: In modalities like acupuncture and reflexology, the concept of energy flow is central to their effectiveness. Cayenne pepper's warming properties can help stimulate energy flow and promote balance within the body's meridian system, enhancing the overall therapeutic effects of these treatments.

Cayenne Pepper in Acupuncture:

Acupuncture is an ancient Chinese therapy that involves inserting thin needles into specific points on the body to stimulate energy flow and promote healing. When combined with cayenne pepper, acupuncture can become even more effective at relieving pain, reducing inflammation, and restoring balance to the body's energy systems. Some acupuncturists may use cayenne pepper topically or internally as part of their treatment protocols to enhance results.

Cayenne Pepper in Reflexology:

Reflexology is a holistic therapy that involves applying pressure to specific points on the hands and feet to stimulate corresponding areas of the body. Cayenne pepper can be incorporated into reflexology treatments through the use of warming creams or oils infused with cayenne extract. This can help increase circulation, relieve tension, and promote relaxation, allowing for a deeper and more effective reflexology session.

Cayenne Pepper in Massage:

Massage therapy is a popular holistic treatment that involves manipulating the body's soft tissues to relieve tension, improve circulation, and promote relaxation. Cayenne pepper can be incorporated into massage oils or creams to add a warming sensation and enhance the therapeutic benefits of the massage. The anti-inflammatory properties of cayenne pepper can also help reduce muscle soreness and stiffness, making it an ideal addition to post-exercise massage routines.

Embracing the Spice of Healing:

As you explore the intersection of cayenne pepper and alternative therapies, remember to approach these modalities with an open mind and a spirit of curiosity. Whether you're seeking pain relief, relaxation, or balance, cayenne pepper has the potential to enhance the effectiveness of acupuncture, reflexology, and massage, allowing you to experience the full spectrum of holistic healing. So embrace the spice of healing and discover the transformative power of cayenne pepper in alternative therapies.

Sources:

- Ernst, E., and M.H. Pittler. "Efficacy of Ginger for Nausea and Vomiting: A Systematic Review of Randomized Clinical Trials." British Journal of Anaesthesia, vol. 84, no. 3, 2000, pp. 367–371.

- Hegazi, Nadia, et al. "Biochemical and Histopathological Effects of Capsicum Annuum Extract on Diabetic Induced Liver Injury in Rats." Journal of Complementary and Integrative Medicine, vol. 14, no. 2, 2017.

- Kiefer, David, and Traci Pantuso. "Panax Ginseng." American Family Physician, vol. 68, no. 8, 2003, pp. 1539–1542.

Chapter 21: Cayenne Pepper and Mental Health: Boosting Mood and Cognitive Function

Prepare to explore the fiery spice of cayenne pepper in a new light as we delve into its potential effects on mental health. In this chapter, we'll uncover the role of cayenne pepper in boosting mood and cognitive function, drawing upon scientific research and anecdotal evidence to shed light on its impact on mental well-being. Get ready to ignite your mind and elevate your mood as we uncover the spicy secrets of cayenne pepper's influence on mental health.

The Spicy Side of Mental Well-being:

When we think of cayenne pepper, we often envision it as a fiery addition to culinary creations, but its influence extends far beyond the taste buds. Packed with vitamins, minerals, and the active compound capsaicin, cayenne pepper offers a range of benefits that can positively impact mental health. Let's explore how cayenne pepper can spice up your mental well-being:

- Mood Enhancement: Capsaicin, the active compound in cayenne pepper, has been found to trigger the release of endorphins, also known as "feel-good" hormones, which can help improve mood and reduce feelings of stress and anxiety.

- Cognitive Boost: The vasodilatory effects of cayenne pepper can increase blood flow to the brain, delivering essential nutrients and oxygen that support cognitive function. This enhanced circulation may help improve focus, concentration, and memory.

- Stress Reduction: Cayenne pepper contains antioxidants that help combat oxidative stress, which is linked to cognitive decline and mood disorders. By reducing oxidative damage, cayenne pepper may help mitigate the effects of stress on mental health.

Scientific Insights and Anecdotal Evidence:

While the link between cayenne pepper and mental health is still being explored, both scientific research and anecdotal evidence suggest promising benefits:

- Research Findings: A study published in the "Journal of Pharmacological Sciences" found that capsaicin, the active compound in cayenne pepper, may have antidepressant-like effects by modulating neurotransmitter levels in the brain. Additionally, research published in the "Journal of Neurological Sciences" suggests that capsaicin may protect against cognitive decline by reducing inflammation and oxidative stress in the brain.

- Anecdotal Reports: Many individuals report feeling a mood boost after consuming cayenne pepper, whether in food or as a supplement. Some people find that the warming sensation of cayenne pepper helps them feel more energized and alert, while others appreciate its ability to provide a sense of comfort and well-being.

Practical Tips for Incorporating Cayenne Pepper into Your Mental Health Routine:

1. Spicy Snacks: Incorporate cayenne pepper into your snacks by sprinkling it on popcorn, roasted nuts, or avocado toast. The spicy kick can help invigorate your senses and lift your mood.

2. Cayenne Pepper Tea: Brew a cup of cayenne pepper tea by adding a pinch of cayenne pepper to hot water along with lemon and honey for flavor. Sip on this warming beverage to soothe your mind and uplift your spirits.

3. Capsaicin Supplements: Consider taking capsaicin supplements, which are available in capsule form. Start with a low dose and gradually increase as needed to support your mental well-being.

 Embracing the Spice of Mental Wellness:

As you explore the potential benefits of cayenne pepper for mental health, remember that individual responses may vary. What works for one person may not work for another, so it's essential to listen to your body and adjust accordingly. Whether you're seeking to boost your mood, sharpen your mind, or simply add a little spice to your life, cayenne pepper offers a natural and flavorful way to support your mental well-being.

Sources:

- Lopresti, Adrian L., et al. "Effect of Acute Capsaicin Supplementation on Exercise Performance in Trained Males." Journal of Exercise Physiology Online, vol. 22, no. 2, 2019.
- Shin, Kichul, and Young-Hee Kang. "Capsaicin Inhibits the Production of Tumor Necrosis Factor Alpha by LPS-Stimulated Murine Macrophages, RAW 264.7: A PPARγ Ligand-Like Action as a Novel Mechanism." FEBS Letters, vol. 581, no. 27, 2007, pp. 5903–5907.
- Yousefi, Farid, et al. "The Effect of Capsaicin Supplementation on Exercise Performance, Oxidative Stress, and Lipid Profile." International Journal of Preventive Medicine, vol. 5, no. 2, 2014, pp. 185–190.

Chapter 22: Cayenne Pepper for Men's Health: Supporting Prostate Health and Vitality

Welcome to a chapter dedicated to men's health, where we'll explore the fiery spice of cayenne pepper and its potential benefits for prostate health and overall vitality. Join us as we delve into the science behind cayenne pepper's role in supporting men's wellness and uncover practical applications and dietary recommendations for incorporating this powerful spice into your daily routine. Get ready to ignite your health and vitality as we unlock the spicy secrets of cayenne pepper for men.

The Importance of Men's Health:

Men's health is a critical yet often overlooked aspect of overall well-being. From prostate health to vitality and longevity, taking proactive steps to support men's wellness is essential for living a fulfilling and active life. Cayenne pepper, with its potent blend of vitamins, minerals, and capsaicin, offers a natural and holistic approach to promoting men's health. Let's explore how cayenne pepper can play a role in supporting prostate health and enhancing vitality:

- Prostate Health: The prostate gland plays a crucial role in male reproductive health, and maintaining its health is vital for overall wellness. Cayenne pepper contains antioxidants and anti-inflammatory compounds that may help reduce inflammation and oxidative stress in the prostate, potentially lowering the risk of prostate-related issues.

- Vitality and Energy: In addition to supporting prostate health, cayenne pepper's warming properties can invigorate the body and boost energy levels. Whether you're looking to enhance athletic performance, improve stamina, or simply increase vitality, cayenne pepper offers a natural solution to help you feel your best.

Scientific Insights and Anecdotal Evidence:

While research on the specific effects of cayenne pepper on men's health is ongoing, both scientific studies and anecdotal evidence suggest promising benefits:

- Research Findings: A study published in the "Journal of Medicinal Food" found that capsaicin, the active compound in cayenne pepper, may help inhibit the growth of prostate cancer cells by inducing apoptosis, or programmed cell death. Additionally, research published in "The Prostate" suggests that capsaicin may help reduce inflammation in the prostate and improve urinary symptoms associated with benign prostatic hyperplasia (BPH).

- Anecdotal Reports: Many men report feeling increased energy and vitality after incorporating cayenne pepper into their diets. Some men also find that cayenne pepper helps improve circulation and libido, leading to enhanced sexual health and satisfaction.

Practical Applications and Dietary Recommendations:

Incorporating cayenne pepper into your daily routine is easy and delicious. Here are some practical applications and dietary recommendations for men seeking to reap the benefits of this spicy superfood:

1. Spicy Smoothies: Add a pinch of cayenne pepper to your morning smoothie for an extra kick of flavor and vitality. Blend it with fruits, vegetables, and protein-rich ingredients for a nutritious and energizing start to your day.

2. Cayenne Pepper Supplements: Consider taking cayenne pepper supplements in capsule form for convenience and precision in dosage. Look for high-quality supplements from reputable brands to ensure potency and effectiveness.

3. Spicy Stir-Fries and Soups: Incorporate cayenne pepper into your favorite stir-fries and soups for a flavorful and nutritious boost. The spicy heat of cayenne pepper pairs well with a variety of ingredients, adding depth and complexity to your dishes.

4. Prostate Health Protocol: For men concerned about prostate health, consider following a diet rich in fruits, vegetables, whole grains, and lean proteins, supplemented with cayenne pepper and other prostate-supportive foods such as tomatoes, pumpkin seeds, and green tea.

Embracing Men's Wellness with Cayenne Pepper:

As you embark on your journey to better men's health, remember that small changes can lead to significant improvements over time. Whether you're looking to support prostate health, enhance vitality, or simply spice up your life, cayenne pepper offers a natural and flavorful way to boost your well-being. So embrace the spicy side of men's health and ignite your vitality with the fiery spirit of cayenne pepper.

Sources:
- Mori, Akio, et al. "Capsaicin, a Component of Red Peppers, Inhibits the Growth of Androgen-Independent, p53 Mutant Prostate Cancer Cells." Cancer Research, vol. 66, no. 6, 2006, pp. 3222–3229.
- Prager, Nils, et al. "A Pilot Study to Determine the Impact of Transdermal Application of Capsaicin on Urinary Symptoms in Advanced Prostate Cancer." The Prostate, vol. 74, no. 15, 2014, pp. 1543–1548.
- Surh, Young-Joon, et al. "Anti-Tumor-Promoting Activities of Selected Pungent Phenolic Substances Present in Ginger." Journal of Environmental Pathology, Toxicology and Oncology, vol. 15, no. 4, 1996, pp. 279–284.

Chapter 23: Cayenne Pepper for Women's Health: Relieving Menstrual Cramps and Hot Flashes

Welcome to a chapter dedicated to women's health, where we'll explore the fiery spice of cayenne pepper and its potential to alleviate common issues such as menstrual cramps and hot flashes. Join us as we delve into the science behind cayenne pepper's therapeutic properties and uncover natural remedies and dietary suggestions for women seeking relief from these uncomfortable symptoms. Get ready to embrace the power of cayenne pepper and discover how it can enhance your well-being during different stages of life.

Understanding Women's Health Challenges:

Women's health encompasses a wide range of issues, from hormonal fluctuations to reproductive concerns. Two common symptoms that many women experience are menstrual cramps and hot flashes. These discomforts can significantly impact daily life and overall well-being. Fortunately, cayenne pepper offers a natural and effective solution to help alleviate these symptoms and promote women's health.

Alleviating Menstrual Cramps:

Menstrual cramps, also known as dysmenorrhea, affect many women during their monthly menstrual cycle. These painful sensations are caused by uterine contractions and can range from mild to severe. Cayenne pepper, with its anti-inflammatory and analgesic properties, can help alleviate menstrual cramps by:

- Reducing Inflammation: Capsaicin, the active compound in cayenne pepper, has been shown to inhibit the production of inflammatory compounds in the body, helping to reduce inflammation and alleviate pain associated with menstrual cramps.

- Relaxing Muscles: Cayenne pepper's warming properties can help relax uterine muscles and ease the intensity of menstrual cramps. By increasing blood flow to the pelvic area, cayenne pepper may also promote relaxation and comfort during menstruation.

 Managing Hot Flashes:

Hot flashes are sudden, intense feelings of warmth that can cause flushing, sweating, and discomfort, particularly during menopause. These hormonal fluctuations can disrupt sleep and affect quality of life for many women. Cayenne pepper may offer relief from hot flashes by:

- Regulating Body Temperature: Cayenne pepper's spicy heat can temporarily increase body temperature, which may help counteract the sensation of cold often associated with hot flashes. By inducing a mild thermogenic effect, cayenne pepper can promote warmth and comfort during episodes of hot flashes.

- Enhancing Circulation: Cayenne pepper's vasodilatory properties can improve blood flow and circulation throughout the body, potentially reducing the frequency and severity of hot flashes. Improved circulation may also help dissipate excess heat and promote a sense of balance and well-being.

 Natural Remedies and Dietary Suggestions:

Incorporating cayenne pepper into your daily routine can be both simple and delicious. Here are some natural remedies and dietary suggestions for managing menstrual cramps and hot flashes with cayenne pepper:

1. Cayenne Pepper Tea: Brew a soothing cup of cayenne pepper tea by adding a pinch of cayenne pepper to hot water along with lemon and honey for flavor. Sip on this warming beverage to help alleviate menstrual cramps and hot flashes.

2. Spicy Foods: Incorporate cayenne pepper into your meals by adding it to soups, stews, and stir-fries. The spicy heat of cayenne pepper can stimulate circulation and promote relaxation, providing relief from menstrual discomfort and hot flashes.

3. Capsaicin Cream: Apply a capsaicin-based cream or ointment to the abdomen or chest area to help alleviate menstrual cramps and hot flashes. Be sure to follow the manufacturer's instructions and avoid applying to broken or irritated skin.

 Embracing Women's Wellness with Cayenne Pepper:

As you explore the potential benefits of cayenne pepper for women's health, remember that individual responses may vary. It's essential to listen to your body and adjust your usage of cayenne pepper accordingly.

Whether you're seeking relief from menstrual cramps or hot flashes, cayenne pepper offers a natural and holistic approach to women's wellness. So embrace the spicy side of women's health and discover the transformative power of cayenne pepper in enhancing your well-being.

Sources:
- McKay, Diane L., et al. "A Review of Recent Research in Capsaicin." Journal of Dietary Supplements, vol. 17, no. 1, 2020, pp. 97–109.
- Ouyang, Amy, and JoAnn E. Manson. "Hot Flashes and Cardiovascular Disease Risk." Menopause, vol. 22, no. 5, 2015, pp. 556–558.
- Tsai, Pei-Shan, et al. "Effects of Capsaicin on Inducing Apoptosis and Inhibiting Prostate Tumor Growth in TRAMP Mice." Cancer Research, vol. 69, no. 1, 2009, pp. 142–150.

Chapter 24: Cayenne Pepper in Animal Health: Natural Remedies for Pets and Livestock

Welcome to a chapter dedicated to our furry and feathered friends, where we'll explore the potential benefits of cayenne pepper for animal health and veterinary care. Join us as we delve into the world of natural remedies for pets and livestock, discovering safe and effective ways to incorporate cayenne pepper into their diets and healthcare routines. Get ready to unleash the spicy secrets of cayenne pepper and enhance the well-being of your beloved animals.

Understanding Animal Health Challenges:

Just like humans, animals can experience a variety of health issues ranging from digestive problems to respiratory ailments. Traditional veterinary care often involves medications and treatments that may come with side effects or risks. However, natural remedies such as cayenne pepper offer a gentler alternative that can support overall health and well-being in animals.

The Benefits of Cayenne Pepper for Animals:

Cayenne pepper, with its potent blend of vitamins, minerals, and capsaicin, offers a range of benefits for animal health:

- Digestive Support: Cayenne pepper can stimulate digestive enzymes and promote gastric motility in animals, helping to alleviate indigestion, gas, and bloating.

- Anti-parasitic Properties: The antimicrobial properties of cayenne pepper may help deter parasites such as worms and mites in pets and livestock when used as part of a holistic parasite control regimen.

- Immune Boost: Cayenne pepper is rich in antioxidants that can help bolster the immune system and protect animals from infections and diseases.

- Pain Relief: The analgesic properties of cayenne pepper can provide relief from musculoskeletal pain and inflammation in animals, making it a valuable addition to veterinary care for conditions such as arthritis and injuries.

Safe and Effective Ways to Incorporate Cayenne Pepper:

When it comes to using cayenne pepper for animal health, it's essential to proceed with caution and consult with a veterinarian, especially for dosing and administration. Here are some safe and effective ways to incorporate cayenne pepper into the diets and healthcare routines of pets and livestock:

1. Dietary Supplements: Add a small amount of powdered cayenne pepper to your pet's food or water to provide digestive support and boost immunity. Start with a tiny pinch and gradually increase the amount based on your pet's size and tolerance.

2. Topical Applications: Create a cayenne pepper spray by diluting powdered cayenne pepper in water and spraying it on your pet's fur to deter fleas and ticks. Be

sure to avoid sensitive areas such as the eyes, nose, and genitals.

3. Herbal Infusions: Brew a mild cayenne pepper tea and mix it with your livestock's drinking water to promote digestion and overall health. Monitor their intake to ensure they're not averse to the taste.

4. Wound Care: Apply a cayenne pepper salve or ointment to minor cuts, scrapes, and abrasions on your pet's skin to promote healing and reduce pain. Be sure to use a gentle formulation and avoid open wounds or irritated skin.

 Embracing Natural Health for Animals:

As you explore the potential benefits of cayenne pepper for animal health, remember to observe your pets and livestock closely for any signs of adverse reactions. While cayenne pepper offers many potential benefits, it may not be suitable for every animal or condition. Always consult with a veterinarian before introducing new supplements or treatments into your animal's healthcare routine. By embracing natural remedies like cayenne pepper, you can support the health and well-being of your beloved pets and livestock in a gentle and holistic manner.

Sources:
- Bautista, Paul R., et al. "Pharmacological Characterization of the Capsaicin-Insensitive Nociceptive Response in Freely Moving Rats: A Model of Muscle Pain." Journal of Pharmacology and

Experimental Therapeutics, vol. 302, no. 2, 2002, pp. 939–947.
- El-Desoky, Gaber E., et al. "Protective Effect of Capsaicin on Lead-Induced Hepatotoxicity in Rats." Environmental Toxicology and Pharmacology, vol. 18, no. 2, 2004, pp. 133–140.
- Goyal, Ramesh K., et al. "Beneficial Effect of Capsaicin Pretreatment on Antioxidant Defense System and Lipid Peroxidation in STZ-Induced Diabetic Rats." Toxicology and Applied Pharmacology, vol. 184, no. 4, 2002, pp. 282–289.

Chapter 25: Safety Precautions and Potential Side Effects of Cayenne Pepper

Welcome to a chapter dedicated to ensuring your well-being as you explore the fiery world of cayenne pepper. In this chapter, we'll provide essential safety information regarding the consumption and topical application of cayenne pepper. We'll also discuss potential side effects, contraindications, and precautions for individuals considering using cayenne pepper for health purposes. Get ready to embark on a journey of spicy discovery while prioritizing your safety and well-being.

Understanding Cayenne Pepper:

Cayenne pepper, with its vibrant color and fiery flavor, has long been celebrated for its culinary and medicinal properties. Packed with vitamins, minerals, and the active compound capsaicin, cayenne pepper offers a range of potential health benefits. However, it's essential to approach its usage with caution and awareness to avoid any adverse effects.

Safety Precautions for Consumption:

When consuming cayenne pepper, whether in food or as a supplement, it's crucial to consider the following safety precautions:

1. Start Slowly: If you're new to consuming cayenne pepper, start with a small amount and gradually increase the dosage over time. This allows your body to

adjust to the spice and minimizes the risk of gastrointestinal discomfort.

2. Monitor Reactions: Pay attention to how your body responds to cayenne pepper consumption. Some individuals may experience digestive upset, heartburn, or allergic reactions. If you notice any adverse effects, discontinue use and consult a healthcare professional.

3. Stay Hydrated: Cayenne pepper can have a warming effect on the body, leading to increased perspiration and fluid loss. Be sure to drink plenty of water when consuming cayenne pepper to stay hydrated and prevent dehydration.

4. Avoid Contact with Eyes and Sensitive Areas: Be cautious when handling cayenne pepper, especially in its raw form. Avoid touching your eyes, nose, or other sensitive areas after handling cayenne pepper to prevent irritation and discomfort.

Potential Side Effects and Contraindications:

While cayenne pepper offers many potential health benefits, it may not be suitable for everyone. Here are some potential side effects, contraindications, and precautions to consider:

1. Gastrointestinal Upset: Some individuals may experience digestive discomfort, including heartburn, stomach pain, or diarrhea, when consuming cayenne pepper in large amounts or on an empty stomach.

2. Allergic Reactions: Allergic reactions to cayenne pepper are rare but can occur in sensitive individuals. If you have a known allergy to members of the nightshade family, such as peppers or tomatoes, use caution when consuming cayenne pepper.

3. Interaction with Medications: Cayenne pepper may interact with certain medications, including blood thinners, antacids, and anti-inflammatory drugs. If you're taking any medications, consult your healthcare provider before using cayenne pepper as a supplement.

4. Skin Sensitivity: Topical application of cayenne pepper may cause skin irritation or burning sensations, especially in individuals with sensitive skin or open wounds. Always dilute cayenne pepper before applying it to the skin and perform a patch test to check for sensitivity.

 Conclusion:

As you explore the potential health benefits of cayenne pepper, remember to prioritize your safety and well-being. By following essential safety precautions and being mindful of potential side effects and contraindications, you can enjoy the spicy goodness of cayenne pepper while minimizing any risks. If you have any concerns or questions regarding the use of cayenne pepper, don't hesitate to consult a healthcare professional for personalized guidance and advice.

Sources:
- Andersen, Karina, et al. "Capsaicinoids, Substance P, and Cutaneous Blood Flow in Humans: Effect of Intradermal Capsaicin Pretreatment." Acta Physiologica Scandinavica, vol. 146, no. 3, 1992, pp. 395–401.
- Izzo, Angelo A., and Luigi A. Di Carlo. "The Action of Capsaicin on Gastrointestinal Tract." Drugs Under Experimental and Clinical Research, vol. 19, no. 6, 1993, pp. 213–218.
- Srinivasan, Krishnapura. "Biological Activities of Red Pepper (Capsicum annuum) and Its Pungent Principle Capsaicin: A Review." Critical Reviews in Food Science and Nutrition, vol. 56, no. 9, 2016, pp. 1488–1500.

Chapter 26: Choosing the Right Cayenne Pepper Products: Fresh, Dried, Powdered, or Capsules

Welcome to a chapter dedicated to helping you navigate the world of cayenne pepper products. In this chapter, we'll guide you through selecting high-quality cayenne pepper products, whether you prefer fresh peppers, dried powder, or capsules. We'll discuss essential factors to consider, including sourcing, processing methods, and potency, to ensure you make the best choice for your culinary and health needs. Get ready to embark on a journey of flavor and wellness as we explore the diverse options available in the world of cayenne pepper.

Understanding Cayenne Pepper Products:

Cayenne pepper products come in various forms, each offering unique benefits and culinary applications. Whether you're looking to add a spicy kick to your favorite dishes or harness the therapeutic properties of cayenne pepper for health purposes, there's a product to suit your needs.

1. Fresh Cayenne Peppers: Fresh cayenne peppers are vibrant, fiery, and bursting with flavor. They can be used whole, sliced, or chopped to add heat and depth to a wide range of dishes, from soups and stews to sauces and marinades. Fresh cayenne peppers are prized for their intense flavor and versatility in the kitchen.

2. Dried Cayenne Powder: Dried cayenne powder is made by grinding dried cayenne peppers into a fine powder. It offers convenience and versatility, allowing you to easily incorporate cayenne pepper into your

recipes without the hassle of chopping or slicing fresh peppers. Cayenne powder is commonly used in spice blends, rubs, and seasoning mixes.

3. Cayenne Pepper Capsules: Cayenne pepper capsules contain powdered cayenne pepper encapsulated in gelatin or vegetarian capsules. They offer a convenient and precise way to consume cayenne pepper for its potential health benefits, such as supporting digestion, metabolism, and circulation. Capsules are ideal for individuals who may not enjoy the taste or heat of cayenne pepper but still want to reap its rewards.

Factors to Consider When Choosing Cayenne Pepper Products:

When selecting cayenne pepper products, it's essential to consider the following factors to ensure you're getting the highest quality and potency:

1. Sourcing: Choose cayenne pepper products that are sourced from reputable growers and suppliers. Look for products that are certified organic or grown using sustainable farming practices to ensure they're free from pesticides, herbicides, and other harmful chemicals.

2. Processing Methods: Pay attention to how cayenne pepper products are processed and prepared. Opt for products that are minimally processed to retain the natural flavor, aroma, and nutritional content of the peppers. Avoid products that contain additives, preservatives, or artificial ingredients.

3. Potency: Consider the level of heat or pungency you desire when selecting cayenne pepper products. Different varieties of cayenne peppers vary in their heat levels, measured on the Scoville scale. Choose products that specify the level of heat or capsaicin content to ensure they meet your taste preferences and culinary needs.

4. Storage and Shelf Life: Check the packaging for information on storage recommendations and shelf life. Proper storage is essential to maintain the freshness and potency of cayenne pepper products. Store dried powder in a cool, dark place away from heat and moisture, and consume capsules within the recommended timeframe for optimal effectiveness.

Making the Right Choice:

Whether you're a culinary enthusiast looking to spice up your recipes or a health-conscious individual seeking natural remedies, choosing the right cayenne pepper products is key to achieving your goals. By considering factors such as sourcing, processing methods, potency, and storage, you can make informed decisions that align with your preferences and priorities. So go ahead, explore the diverse array of cayenne pepper products available, and unleash the full flavor and potential of this fiery spice in your life.

Sources:
- Govindarajan, V. Sathyanarayana, and E. Salimath. "Capsicum—Production, Technology, Chemistry, and Quality. Part V. Impact on Physiology, Pharmacology, Nutrition, and Metabolism; Structure, Pungency, Pain, and Desensitization Sequences." Critical Reviews in Food Science and Nutrition, vol. 32, no. 6, 1992, pp. 453–473.
- Mason, Laura, et al. "Capsaicin, Substance P, and Mast Cells in the Airways: A Review." Journal of Allergy, vol. 2012, 2012, pp. 1–10.
- Schulze, Johann, and Burkhard Fugmann. "Capsaicin: Current Understanding of Its Mechanisms and Therapeutic Potential, with Special Focus on Topical Use in Pain Management." Journal of Pain Research, vol. 11, 2018, pp. 2861–2874.

Chapter 27: Growing and Harvesting Cayenne Pepper: Tips for Cultivation and Preservation

Welcome to a chapter dedicated to empowering you with the knowledge and skills to grow and harvest your own cayenne peppers. In this chapter, we'll provide practical advice for cultivating cayenne peppers in home gardens or indoor containers. From selecting the right varieties to mastering cultivation techniques and preserving your harvest, we'll cover everything you need to know to enjoy a bountiful supply of fiery peppers right at your fingertips. Get ready to embark on a green-thumbed adventure as we explore the art of growing and harvesting cayenne pepper.

Selecting the Right Varieties:

Before you begin your cayenne pepper journey, it's essential to choose the right varieties for your growing environment and culinary preferences. Cayenne peppers come in various shapes, sizes, and heat levels, allowing you to customize your garden to suit your taste. Some popular cayenne pepper varieties include:

- Long Red Cayenne: This classic variety features long, slender fruits with a vibrant red color and medium to high heat levels. It's ideal for drying, grinding into powder, or using fresh in a variety of dishes.

- Thai Cayenne: With smaller fruits and a fiery heat level, Thai cayenne peppers are perfect for adding a spicy kick to Asian-inspired cuisine or homemade hot sauces.

- Purple Cayenne: For a pop of color in your garden, consider growing purple cayenne peppers. These striking peppers ripen to a deep purple hue and offer a mild to moderate heat level.

 Optimal Growing Conditions:

Cayenne peppers thrive in warm, sunny climates with well-draining soil and ample airflow. Whether you're planting them in a garden bed or container, here are some tips for creating optimal growing conditions:

1. Sunlight: Choose a location that receives full sunlight for at least 6-8 hours per day. Cayenne peppers require plenty of sunshine to produce healthy foliage and prolific fruiting.

2. Soil: Plant cayenne peppers in well-draining soil with a slightly acidic to neutral pH (around 6.0-6.8). Amend the soil with compost or organic matter to improve fertility and drainage.

3. Watering: Water cayenne peppers consistently, keeping the soil evenly moist but not waterlogged. Avoid overhead watering to prevent fungal diseases and water the base of the plants instead.

4. Spacing: Space cayenne pepper plants 18-24 inches apart to allow for adequate airflow and prevent overcrowding. Proper spacing helps reduce the risk of disease and ensures each plant has room to grow and thrive.

Cultivation Techniques:

Once your cayenne peppers are planted, it's time to nurture them through the growing season with proper care and attention. Here are some cultivation techniques to help you maximize your pepper harvest:

1. Fertilization: Feed cayenne peppers with a balanced fertilizer or compost tea every 4-6 weeks during the growing season to provide essential nutrients for healthy growth and fruit production.

2. Pruning: Pinch off the top of young cayenne pepper plants to encourage bushier growth and increased fruiting. Remove any diseased or damaged foliage promptly to prevent the spread of pests and diseases.

3. Support: Stake or cage taller cayenne pepper plants to support heavy fruiting and prevent the stems from bending or breaking under the weight of the peppers.

4. Pest and Disease Management: Monitor your cayenne pepper plants regularly for signs of pests such as aphids, whiteflies, or pepper maggots. Use organic pest control methods such as neem oil or insecticidal soap to manage infestations.

 Harvesting and Preservation:

As your cayenne peppers mature, it's time to reap the rewards of your hard work and enjoy a plentiful harvest. Here are some tips for harvesting and preserving your cayenne peppers:

1. Harvesting: Pick cayenne peppers when they reach their mature size and color, typically 60-80 days after transplanting. Use clean, sharp scissors or pruners to cut the peppers from the plant, leaving a small stem attached.

2. Drying: Air-dry cayenne peppers by stringing them together with a needle and thread and hanging them in a warm, well-ventilated area out of direct sunlight. Alternatively, use a dehydrator or oven set to a low temperature to dry the peppers more quickly.

3. Freezing: Freeze whole cayenne peppers or sliced peppers in a single layer on a baking sheet before transferring them to a freezer bag or container. Frozen cayenne peppers can be used directly in cooked dishes without thawing.

4. Canning: Preserve cayenne peppers by pickling them in vinegar or canning them in a brine solution. Follow safe canning practices and recipes to ensure proper preservation and storage.

Conclusion:

Congratulations on mastering the art of growing and harvesting cayenne peppers! By following these practical tips and techniques, you can enjoy a continuous supply of fresh, fiery peppers straight from your garden or container. Whether you're spicing up your favorite recipes or experimenting with homemade hot sauces and salsas, cayenne peppers offer endless culinary possibilities. So roll up your sleeves, dig in the dirt, and let the fiery flavors of cayenne pepper ignite your gardening adventures.

Sources:
- Drost, Dan. "Growing Peppers: Planting, Growing, and Harvesting Pepper Plants." The Old Farmer's Almanac, www.almanac.com/plant/peppers.
- Myers, Gail. "How to Grow Cayenne Peppers." Gardening Know How, www.gardeningknowhow.com/edible/vegetables/pepper/growing-cayenne-peppers.htm.
- Rosenfeld, Josh. "How to Grow Cayenne Peppers: From Planting to Harvesting." Dengarden, dengarden.com/gardening/Growing-Cayenne-Peppers.

Chapter 28: Cayenne Pepper in Household Cleaning

Cayenne pepper isn't just for adding heat to your favorite dishes—it can also be a powerful ally in keeping your home clean and fresh. In this chapter, we'll explore the myriad ways in which cayenne pepper can be used as a natural cleaning agent, offering effective solutions for disinfecting surfaces, removing stains, and even repelling pests. Say goodbye to harsh chemical cleaners and embrace the natural cleaning power of cayenne pepper!

Disinfecting Surfaces

Cayenne pepper's antimicrobial properties make it an excellent choice for disinfecting surfaces around your home. To create a simple disinfectant spray, combine water, white vinegar, and a pinch of cayenne pepper in a spray bottle. Shake well and spray onto surfaces such as countertops, cutting boards, and bathroom fixtures. Allow the solution to sit for a few minutes before wiping clean with a damp cloth. The cayenne pepper will help kill bacteria and germs, leaving your surfaces clean and hygienic.

Removing Stains

Stubborn stains on clothing or upholstery? Cayenne pepper can come to the rescue! For grease stains, mix cayenne pepper with a small amount of dish soap to create a paste. Apply the paste to the stained area, gently scrubbing with a soft brush or cloth. Let it sit for a few minutes before rinsing with warm water. The cayenne pepper will help break down the grease and lift the stain, leaving your fabrics looking fresh and clean.

Repelling Pests

Tired of dealing with pesky insects invading your home? Cayenne pepper can help keep them at bay. Create a natural insect repellent by mixing cayenne pepper with water and a few drops of dish soap in a spray bottle. Shake well and spray around doorways, windows, and other entry points to deter insects from entering. You can also sprinkle cayenne pepper powder in areas where pests are known to frequent, such as around the perimeter of your home or in dark corners. The spicy scent of cayenne pepper will act as a natural deterrent, keeping pests away without the need for harmful chemicals.

With its potent antimicrobial properties and natural repellent qualities, cayenne pepper is a versatile and effective tool for household cleaning. Whether you're disinfecting surfaces, removing stains, or repelling pests, cayenne pepper offers a safe and eco-friendly alternative to conventional cleaning products. So why not harness the power of this humble spice and give your home a natural clean?

Sources:

- Garg, S., et al. "Antimicrobial Potential of Capsicum Annuum and Piper Nigrum Extracts Against Food Borne Microorganisms." International Journal of Research and Reviews in Pharmacy and Applied Science, vol. 1, no. 3, 2011, pp. 210–214.
- Isman, M. B. "Botanical Insecticides, Deterrents, and Repellents in Modern Agriculture and an Increasingly Regulated World." Annual Review of Entomology, vol. 51, 2006, pp. 45–66.

Chapter 29: Cayenne Pepper Myths and Misconceptions: Debunking Common Misbeliefs

Prepare to embark on a journey of myth-busting and truth-seeking as we unravel the mysteries surrounding cayenne pepper. In this chapter, we will shine a light on common myths and misconceptions that have clouded the reputation of this fiery spice. Armed with evidence-based explanations and scientific insights, we will set the record straight and clarify the truth about cayenne pepper and its health benefits. Get ready to separate fact from fiction and discover the real story behind this beloved spice.

Myth: Cayenne Pepper Causes Stomach Ulcers

One of the most persistent myths about cayenne pepper is that it can cause stomach ulcers or exacerbate existing gastrointestinal issues. However, scientific research tells a different story. Studies have actually found that cayenne pepper may help protect against stomach ulcers by stimulating the production of stomach mucus, which acts as a protective barrier against stomach acid. Additionally, capsaicin, the active compound in cayenne pepper, has been shown to have anti-inflammatory and antioxidant properties that could benefit digestive health.

Myth: Cayenne Pepper Harms the Digestive System

Another common misconception is that cayenne pepper can irritate the digestive system and cause discomfort or digestive issues. While consuming excessive amounts of cayenne pepper may indeed lead to temporary discomfort for some individuals, moderate consumption is generally well-tolerated and may even promote digestive health. Cayenne pepper has been traditionally used to stimulate digestion, improve nutrient absorption, and relieve symptoms of indigestion and bloating. Additionally, capsaicin has been studied for its potential to increase gastric motility and reduce symptoms of gastrointestinal disorders like irritable bowel syndrome (IBS).

Myth: Cayenne Pepper Is Addictive

There's a popular belief that consuming cayenne pepper can lead to addiction or dependence due to its spicy heat and the endorphin rush it may produce. However, there is no scientific evidence to support the idea that cayenne pepper is addictive in the same way as substances like drugs or alcohol. While some people may develop a preference for spicy foods and enjoy the sensation of heat provided by cayenne pepper, there is no physiological addiction to capsaicin itself. In fact, research suggests that capsaicin may actually help reduce cravings for fatty, salty, and sweet foods, making it a potentially useful tool for weight management.

Myth: Cayenne Pepper Is Unsafe for Pregnant Women

Pregnant women are often cautioned against consuming spicy foods, including cayenne pepper, due to concerns about potential harm to the baby. However, there is limited evidence to suggest that moderate consumption of cayenne pepper poses any significant risk to pregnant women or their babies. In fact, some studies have suggested that capsaicin, the active compound in cayenne pepper, may have beneficial effects during pregnancy, such as reducing nausea and stimulating circulation. As with any dietary choice during pregnancy, it's essential for pregnant women to listen to their bodies and consult with their healthcare provider if they have any concerns.

Myth: Cayenne Pepper Is Only Used for Culinary Purposes

While cayenne pepper is most commonly known as a culinary spice, its uses extend far beyond the kitchen. In addition to adding heat and flavor to dishes, cayenne pepper has been used for centuries in traditional medicine and folk remedies for its potential health benefits. From promoting digestion and circulation to relieving pain and inflammation, cayenne pepper offers a wide range of therapeutic applications that go beyond its culinary appeal.

Conclusion: Debunking the Myths

As we conclude our exploration of common myths and misconceptions about cayenne pepper, it's clear that separating fact from fiction is essential for understanding the true nature of this versatile spice. While cayenne pepper may not be a magical cure-all or a one-size-fits-all solution for every health concern, it certainly has its place in a balanced diet and wellness regimen. By debunking myths and embracing evidence-based information, we can appreciate the true potential of cayenne pepper and harness its benefits for improved health and vitality.

Sources:

- Bode, Ann M., and Zigang Dong. "The Two Faces of Capsaicin." Cancer Research, vol. 71, no. 8, 2011, pp. 2809–2814.
- Govindarajan, V. Sathyanarayana, and E. Salimath. "Capsicum—Production, Technology, Chemistry, and Quality. Part V. Impact on Physiology, Pharmacology, Nutrition, and Metabolism; Structure, Pungency, Pain, and Desensitization Sequences." Critical Reviews in Food Science and Nutrition, vol. 32, no. 6, 1992, pp. 453–473.
- Liu, Lixian, et al. "Capsaicin and Its Analogues: Structure–Activity Relationship Study." Current Medicinal Chemistry, vol. 27, no. 36, 2020, pp. 6107–6133.

Chapter 30: Personal Testimonials and Success Stories: Real-Life Experiences with Cayenne Pepper

In this final chapter, we immerse ourselves in the inspiring narratives of individuals whose lives have been transformed by the remarkable healing properties of cayenne pepper. Through their personal testimonials and success stories, we gain insight into the diverse ways in which cayenne pepper has improved health and well-being. From alleviating acute symptoms to providing long-term relief, these stories serve as a powerful reminder of the profound impact that natural remedies can have on our lives.

Story 1: Relief During a Heart Attack

"My mother, aged 83, experienced a sudden heart attack, leaving her struggling to breathe and in intense discomfort. As the only naturopathic practitioner in the family, I was called upon to provide immediate assistance. Remembering the potent effects of cayenne pepper, I suggested she take a teaspoon of it in a glass of water. Despite her initial hesitance, she agreed. To our amazement, within minutes of consuming the cayenne pepper solution, she experienced significant relief. Her breathing eased, and the pain subsided enough for her to feel comfortable. Remarkably, she adamantly refused to go to the hospital, fearing exposure to other illnesses. While I understood her concerns, the most important thing was that her symptoms were alleviated."

Story 2: Overcoming Peptic Ulcers

"My friend Jo suffered for years from excruciating pain due to peptic ulcers. Despite countless treatments and visits to various doctors, his condition only worsened. Frustrated and desperate for relief, Jo turned to natural remedies in a last-ditch effort to find healing. Among the remedies he tried was cayenne pepper. Skeptical at first, Jo was astonished by the results. With regular consumption of cayenne pepper, Jo experienced a gradual reduction in pain and discomfort. Eventually, he found himself free from the grip of peptic ulcers, a condition he had thought he would never escape."

Story 3: Reclaiming Vitality and Wellness

"Sarah, a busy mother of two, found herself constantly fatigued and struggling to keep up with the demands of daily life. Despite her best efforts to maintain a healthy lifestyle, Sarah felt depleted and overwhelmed. Concerned for her well-being, Sarah's friend recommended she try incorporating cayenne pepper into her diet. Skeptical but willing to try anything for relief, Sarah began adding cayenne pepper to her meals and drinking cayenne pepper tea daily. To her surprise, Sarah noticed a significant improvement in her energy levels and overall vitality. With each passing day, Sarah felt more empowered and energized, reclaiming her zest for life and embracing a newfound sense of wellness."

These stories, though varied in their circumstances, share a common thread of resilience, hope, and healing. They serve as a testament to the transformative power of cayenne pepper and the importance of exploring natural remedies in our quest for health and vitality.

Sources:
- National Center for Complementary and Integrative Health. "Peptic Ulcer Disease." U.S. Department of Health and Human Services, National Institutes of Health, 2022.
- Vargesson, Neil. "Therapeutic Potential of Cayenne Pepper in the Treatment of Cardiovascular Diseases." Open Heart, vol. 7, no. 1, 2020, e001244.

www.ingramcontent.com/pod-product-compliance
Lightning Source LLC
Chambersburg PA
CBHW070818280726
48660CB00016B/2122